This book belor

If found, please contact me at:

mithmoth

Made in the USA
Las Vegas, NV
22 May 2023

72373511R00072